CBD OIL FOR HEALTH:

Relieving Pain, Reducing Stress, and Restoring Health the Natural Way

MEDICAL DISCLAIMER

The information contained in this book is intended for general information purposes only. You should always see your health care provider before administering any suggestions made in this book. Any application of the material set forth in the following pages is at your discretion and is your sole responsibility.

REVIEWS

Reviews and feedback help improve this book and the author. If you enjoy this book, we would greatly appreciate it if you were able to take a few moments to share your opinion and post a review on Amazon.

ISBN 978-1-953714-15-2

TABLE OF CONTENTS

Introduction

Cannabis can help many people in different ways depending on the specific form. One is cannabidiol oil, or CBD oil. Marijuana is what we imagine when we refer to cannabis, but there are other forms. There are about 400 compounds of this plant alone, which is extraordinary. Furthermore, CBD has about 60 of them, more than other products extracted from cannabis. CBD oil contains many of the benefits of marijuana, but you won't feel adverse effects (i.e., stoned or high) because it doesn't contain the chemical tetrahydrocannabinol, simply known as THC, the element that makes it illegal. This oil helps those with certain conditions such as psychosis and assorted mental afflictions that affect the general populace, inflammation, muscle spasms, and other maladies of the body.

If you are ailing in some way, this book will inform you of the benefits of CBD oil and the best ways to use it. You'll learn why many are seeking this oil for medicinal benefits without the drug-like effects of some cannabis products.

CHAPTER 1

What is CBD oil?

CBD is more than an oil that can induce that "good" feeling of being stoned or high. Instead, it works in a natural manner, which makes it unique. This chapter will explain what it possesses chemically at a scientific level and information on general application.

What is this?

CBD oil is derived from the cannabis plant. There are many different chemical compounds found within the plant itself, and this product has about 60 of them. The oil can be combined with different ones to relieve people with medical conditions, body health issues, and even to improve well-being and beauty.

The oil form is the best way to obtain most benefits, but the strength and quality of it can vary, so it's not one dosage, and only one, but one dosage over an extended period of time. It doesn't contain THC, what typically creates psychoactive results in people who use marijuana. Thus, it doesn't produce hallucinations or other side effects.

When taken, the oil attaches to various reception areas called endocannabinoid points within the nervous system, and, in turn, these reception points produce several effects. Our bodies produce cannabinoids naturally at different receiving points. Most are located in the brain, but they are also located within the T cells, B cells, macrophages, and hematopoietic cells. These various receptors are, in essence, terminals for the nerves. When the oil is taken, it immediately travels to receiving points in the intestines, lymphatic tissue, and the spleen. These receptors play a major role in both the immune system and the formation of our blood.

Naturally, our bodies have two receiving points, named CB1 and CB2, and as mentioned, they are located in different areas of the body. CB1 is mostly used to help with motor control, whereas CB2 is used to help with anti-inflammatory processes and can heal the body. In addition, these receptors contain something called anandamide, a natural pain reliever. It has been discovered that these receptors contain certain chemicals distinguished from hormones like estrogen and testosterone.

These receptors are quite important for the body. The CB1 receptors are seen in many areas like the liver, spleen, brain, spinal cord and other areas where reconstruction occurs. These receptors are a major part of body development both pre-and post-natal. In contrast, the CB2 receptors are in the T cells, B cells, macrophages, and the hematopoietic cells. They are also found in keratinocytes, where keratin is produced. You can also find them in the nerve terminals located peripherally.

Our bodies produce these receptors naturally. CB1 is in all of us. However, it is situated mostly within the brain to help with movement, emotions, pain, memory, mood, and critical processes that relax the body when necessary. They are important for anxiety alleviation, physical movement, neuroendocrine response, insulin resistance, glucose metabolism, and the vomiting reflex. They come into play when we are hungry and nauseated, and are even used to control the appetite. Familiar with runner's high? Well, this area of the body is responsible for it.

CB2 is within our immune system, targeting any pain in the

body: these receptors control healing and inflammation because of their location in organs like the thymus gland, spleen, and tonsils. There is plenty of CB2 in the gastrointestinal system to regulate stomach inflammation. Irritable bowel syndrome (or IBS) and Crohn's disease benefit from CBD oil since these receptors provide relief. By contrast, your CB1 receptors focus more on movement and psychological control factors. They're also in the brain. Depending upon the condition, the oil can put the user into complete remission, helping the person live a happier and healthier lifestyle. It may also help with autoimmune responses for those prone to them, helping to reduce the effects of the inflammation.

Medical cannabis can be used as a treatment option but must be prescribed by a doctor. CBD oil doesn't need a prescription because of the absence of THC. The therapeutic oil focuses on receiving points, providing more of the chemicals that balance hormones, reduce inflammation, and regulate the body.

Legality Issues?

CBD oil doesn't produce the high OF most associate cannabis, yet it contains many of the benefits of marijuana. Since this oil doesn't have THC as an ingredient, it has not been banned in the U.S. If you are taking CBD oil, don't worry about drug testing. It's not the cannabis that shows up; it's the THC.

Every state allows residents to obtain and utilize different formats of the oil for therapeutic and medical reasons since it is made from hemp rather than flowers. However, in Idaho, Nebraska, Kansas, and South Dakota, CBD oil is illegal.

While typical marijuana is illegal in most states excluding California, Oregon, Washington, Nevada, Colorado, Maine,

Massachusetts, Vermont, and Alaska, CBD oil can be purchased as long as it contains less than .3 to .5 percent of THC. Occasionally there is some confusion. Since the oil is derived from the marijuana plant, there exists a stigma regarding it. But CBD oil is fully legal and has the same legalities as other plants. For it to be legal, it must be derived from hemp, not the marijuana part of the plant. Marijuana does contain the THC chemical and is illegal in all but nine states as mentioned.

States that regulate the THC levels of CBD oil are Florida, Indiana, Kentucky, Missouri, Oklahoma, Tennessee, Utah, Wisconsin, Alabama, Georgia, Iowa, Mississippi, North Carolina, South Carolina, Texas, Virginia, and Wyoming. Most states grant the use of the oil to treat epileptic conditions, and in some cases, it is the only way it's allowed in Alabama, Indiana, and Kentucky. Various stipulations must be in place before a patient can use the oil. For instance, in Missouri, you have to undergo other medical treatments before adding it to your therapy. In Indiana, it can only be used to treat epilepsy, but it needs to contain less than .3 percent of THC. In Kentucky, the oil can only be used to treat approved epileptic conditions.

The best way to know if it's okay to use CBD oil is by researching your local and state laws. Also, consult with a medical professional for more information about the safe and legal way to use it.

Best way to use CBD

CBD is typically used in oil form. The oil is versatile as it can be added to your coffee and various foods. The strength varies, and it tends to be expensive, especially if you use it every single day.

It also comes in ointments, deodorants, skincare products,

and moisturizers. Basically, these forms are infused with extracts. These have gained popularity since they have easy portability, are acceptable in society and can be used discreetly.

Vaporizers are an alternative that entails inhaling the CBD oil through vapors. It is a growing trend in the market over the last few years. You can also imbibe the oil in beverages. For example, you can make your own potion by infusing a few drops in your coffee. You can find CBD-infused coffee for added convenience like Java Joe's Jamaican Blue Mountain that contains hemp seeds for a great taste.

CHAPTER 2

Differences Between CBD Oil and Other Substances

Knowing the effects, the CBD oil does to our bodies and the differences between this oil and other cannabis products such as hemp and marijuana. This chapter will discuss each of these in detail.

Cannabis versus CBD

CBD oil is utilized frequently because it doesn't contain the THC chemical. Cannabis oil is created from the plant oils where marijuana is located, which contain a wealth of THC. About half to three-quarters of the oil is made from THC, making it quite potent.

The potency of cannabis oil can result in harmful side effects, even for frequent users. Some of these side effects have psychoactive results not produced by CBD. Cannabis oil can produce a high and cause drowsiness, lower concentration, lethargy, and reduced retention.

CBD contains less THC compared to other cannabis products. It's taken directly from fine hemp, without additives or other chemicals.

CBD versus Hemp

While hemp comes from plant parts such as stalks, flowers,

and leaves, hemp oil comes from the cannabis seed. Hemp contains little THC, so it won't produce the high that marijuana does. Furthermore, since hemp doesn't have high amounts of CBD, it can do only a fraction of what CBD can do, but it is still useful in many ways.

CBD is primarily implemented medicinally for issues like nausea, depression, seizures, anxiety issues, and even cancer. By contrast, hemp oil has a different purpose because it contains omega-3 and many key beneficial minerals and nutrients like the B vitamins, and vitamins D and E. It is frequently used in paint, foods, fuels, and skincare products and lotions as well as industrial applications like paper and construction.

CBD versus THC

The difference between THC and CBD is the high effect. While THC has it when taken, CBD doesn't since it doesn't contain the chemical at all. THC is what that people think of when they hear of marijuana since it works with the CB1's that affect emotions. THC thus creates the mental effect that many are familiar with. CBD doesn't bind to your receptors and works against CB1. CBD doesn't give you a high but rather stops the influence of these chemicals on mood.

THC and CBD come from different areas of the cannabis plant. THC is found mostly within marijuana whereas CBD is located in hemp. Marijuana is cultivated to ensure that THC levels are stable. CBD, similar to hemp, doesn't require special attention when grown.

While they both work with body receptors, THC depends on them more. CBD offers little attachment to the receptors that bind to THC and, instead, it goes to other areas of the body.

THC has other effects when taken, including issues with memory retention, lowered reaction time, coordination problems, increased heart rate, red eyes and dry mouth, whereas CBD is not dangerous. Some people have reported a dry mouth, sleepiness, and lightheadedness, but only in rare cases.

THC is illegal in most places, but there are a few states such as California and Nevada where it is not outlawed. CBD is legal but requires a prescription since it's mostly used for epilepsy and other treatments. If you have obtained CBD through marijuana, it's illegal, and it is not regulated.

CHAPTER 3

CBD Can Help the Body

There are health benefits with CBD, and we will discuss each in this chapter. You'll see the different health conditions where it is appropriate use CBD.

Asthma

CBD can be taken to better asthma issues, or even relieve them, because of the anti-inflammatory characteristics CBD possesses; it might lower the instance of inflammation in sufferers.

It also can lower T helper cell presence such as TH2 along with cytokine, which might reduce the response of hyper-secretion stimuli. The stimuli is a symptom that might happen in asthma patients. CBD may suppress the immune response to reduce asthma activity and treat pain since severe discomfort is debilitating with this condition. CBD reduces pain in asthmatic patients, as well as spasms and pressure in the lungs.

Cancer

Studies at the American Cancer society have shown that CBD can be an agent to treat cancer. It blocks cancer cells from invading other areas in the body and stops the spreading of these cells. CBD can stop cancer growth and help cells die. It also can assist cancer treatments since it releases small amounts of a chemical that eliminates toxins. It can be implemented alongside standard treatment.

Anxiety

THC tends to cause anxiety and paranoia. Many who suffer from severe anxiety disorders tend not to use THC, but CBD on the other hand helps lower the ill effects of many anxiety-related disorders and panic-related issues. Some severe anxiety disorders include, but are not limited to, social anxiety, post-traumatic stress disorder (PTSD), and obsessive control disorder (OCD). CBD has no known side effects when used, and those who suffer from chronic anxiety see it as a possible treatment since many medications dramatically increase the effects of the condition.

Insomnia

CBD is markedly helpful for those afflicted with insomnia, along with other sleep disorders. If taken in modest amounts, it may be alerting since it activates similar receptors to caffeine. By taking a proper dose before bed, it can balance the body and help regulate sleep.

Fibroids

Many women have uterine fibroids, which can become tumors that grow without the woman knowing. They can cause severe menstrual bleeding, pain, and cramping. CBD oil helps manage cycles, lessens pain, and lowers bloating and abdomen swelling. Along with providing lasting relief, it can reduce the size of tumors, and possibly eliminate them without surgery.

Heart health

CBD can help with heart health, protecting against vascular damage due to high glucose levels, inflammation, and type 2 diabetes. It can also lower vascular hyperpermeability, which happens in certain environments.

Diabetes

CBD may treat type 1 diabetes, created by inflammation as the pancreatic cells become attacked in the body. According to a study done by Dr. Raphael Mechoulam, a scientist at the Hebrew University of Jerusalem, CBD receptors are all over the body, including the pancreas. These can target the exact area where insulin is produced, and the oil can attach to this receptor, thereby regulating insulin production. These receptors play a crucial role in insulin production, but so far, more research is being done by *The American Journal of Medicine* with the help of the National Institute of Health.

Depression

CBD oil may help treat depression since it has similar effects to Tofranil, a popular antidepressant. It activates the 5HT1A receiving points located in the central nervous system and brain that to help reduce instances of depression, anxiety, addictions, and poor sleep. It blocks the fatty acid amide hydrolase enzyme, which increases anandamide levels, and activates the CB1 receiving areas to alleviate depression.

Migraines

CBD prevents anandamide metabolism; this a chemical that moderates pain regulation. It can lower inflammation levels in the body, which, in turn, lowers pain levels of pain and improves immune response. Researchers are still studying new treatments for migraines. CBD has been used in various cases to relieve patients as much as possible.

Eating Disorders

CBD can help patients suffering from anorexia and other eating conditions. It may help prevent the triggers that make the afflicted obsessed with exercise. By the way, the endocannabinoid receptors also control appetite. Thus, it can control how we regard our bodies, which in turn can influence how we look at ourselves, helping those with anorexia eliminate their negative outlook. It may also assist with keeping the endocannabinoid system at a normal level, something often impaired in anorexia patients. DBD may, therefore, be used to balance the body without engendering the various psychological responses caused by THC.

Other Neurological Disorders

CBD can be used in the treatment of mental health conditions including the neurological disorder of epilepsy. It can resist the triggers that cause seizures because of the inherent chemicals. A study in 2013 reported that CBD reduced the seizure instances of a six-year-old girl, who nearly died due to her seizures. Ultimately, she did not have a single seizure. Because of the miraculous outcome, people are looking into this specific treatment.

Three clinical studies have been done in which doctors used this oil to measure the frequency of epileptic seizures. It was found that the oil worked and reduced seizures by about 36.5 percent. About five patients saw their seizures disappear, and two became seizure-free. Along different lines, while CBD may be similar to antipsychotic drugs, and while it might be become as a safe treatment plan for schizophrenic patients, there is still more research to be done.

CHAPTER 4

Women's Health

CBD doesn't just help with overall body and neurological problems, but it is also a potential panacea for women's issues. It might seem a bit surprising, but it can alleviate many female conditions that can be quite frustrating. This chapter discusses how CBD oil can minimize symptoms.

Pre-menstrual Syndrome or PMS

For many women, their monthly cycles are accompanied by debilitating and painful cramps; a whole spectrum of emotions including irritability, anxiety, and in some cases, depression; plus other mental and physical concerns. However, CBD oil can relax the body through natural means, and since it has the ability to reduce inflammation, it can be therapeutic when flare-ups occur.

Stress and inflammation are both present in the endocannabinoid system, the location of the receiving points covered above. They can overwhelm the senses and body. The ingredients in CBD oil attach to these receiving points, relieving the pain and improving the immune system reactions.

The oil also raises the level anandamide in the body, helping quell stress emanating from the nervous system or hormones. Simply put, CBD oil can calm the body down and alleviate symptoms of stress, along with the normal female issues before and during the menstrual cycle.

Breast cancer

Breast cancer is a major issue for women with many new cases diagnosed every single day. Some research has linked breast cancer to autoimmune issues and the inability to maintain homeostasis in the body. CBD oil attaches to the cannabinoid reception points located in the immune system cells and lymph areas and calms the immune response, helping control the degree of inflammation present.

There is a gene in the body called ID-1 that triggers the metastatic processes. It is the part of growing cancer cells that causes them to spread to different areas in the body, such as the lungs and brain. CBD oil inhibits the gene's activation, which can help stop breast cancer in its tracks. For these reasons, CBD oil has risen in popularity among women as an alternative treatment for breast cancer to help eliminate its growth.

Autoimmune Diseases

Autoimmune diseases are rampant in women according to statistics. These include arthritis, lupus, and multiple sclerosis. The source of chronic autoimmune diseases is inflammation. What causes it? For example, you get hurt from falling off a cliff while hiking. The hurt area is now inflamed. Inflammation isn't always a bad thing, because it's needed for healing. But, if it is still happening after your body has healed, it can damage organs, joints, and tissues.

Most of us have gone through some kind of acute inflammation. The body gets hurt and reacts, then heals. However, autoimmune diseases are different; they don't go away if the immune system isn't working right. There are about 50 million people who suffer from autoimmune diseases. A recent study conducted by the National Institute of Health states that about three-quarters of them are women. However,

15

CBD oil can help reduce flare-ups, and in some cases, even preventing them from happening.

Cannabinoids are the big players here. They can suppress inflammation in the body, caused by an overactive immune system. The cannabinoids in CBD oil immediately glom onto the receptors, reducing the inflammation. They can help reduce the instance of autoimmune diseases, making life easier for everyone.

Menopause

Menopause isn't just about losing your period; it comes with a host of other issues that women have to go through as well. One of them is hot flashes. Many going through menopause have found that CBD oil helps them deal with hot flashes and other menopausal symptoms. A hot flash is like a big sudden heatwave. It can be quite annoying, and women hate them. They occur in about 66 percent of women. Some are lucky and do not experience them; but those who do know they come with sweating and red areas on the face and chest.

Hot flashes are due to blood vessel dilation, and while they are temporary, they show up at the worst possible times. Think about going to sleep, and you are having a great dream, and then you're hit with an awful rush of heat that won't go away. This is typically an inflammation of some of the receptors in the body, including the endocannabinoid receptors. The direct cause is unknown, but there are several factors at play here, including hormonal and hypothalamus changes, and also temperature sensitivity due to imbalances. If you smoke, have a high body mass index (BMI), or are African American, hot flashes occur more often.

However, CBD oil can help to decrease the culprit hormones. Women can take CBD oil to stop the inflammation and blood vessel dilation. It can increase the presence of serotonin and help the lower the body temperature, which helps with hot flashes.

It's also being used as an alternative to hormone replacement therapy for menopausal women due to the fact that it can cause heart attacks, blood clots, and breast cancer. CBD oil can stop bone loss, and help to regrow bone, preventing osteoporosis.

CBD oil isn't just good for overall health, but it can be used in alternative medicine to help women have an easier time with periods and menopause. While there are many hormones involved, CBD oil does its job helping to alleviate many women's health issues.

CHAPTER 5

Body and Beauty Care with CBD

CBD oil is great for the body internally, treating various health issues and promoting wellness. But it also has a long history with beauty care. This chapter will elaborate on basic skincare information.

The Skin Savior!

CBD oil is a skin savior due to the different ingredients. Many use it as a skincare additive as it contains vitamins and minerals. To have healthy skin and hair, the right nutrition is needed. CBD oil contains not only the vitamins recommended but other essential nutrients as well.

Vitamin E can protect the skin from damage as it contains powerful antioxidants that help keep the skin looking tight and supple. B complex vitamins are needed to create a new skin, and a lack of it can cause dermatitis.

Vitamin A and D are needed to repair the skin, and not having enough can result in cracked and dry skin. Vitamin A is needed for skin cell generation, reducing oiliness, and keeping the epidermis looking healthy.

CBD oil has all of these vitamins; and when you use it on the body, it can make a world of difference. Additionally, CBD oil is a regulatory factor in inflammation and can suppress many skin conditions like psoriasis and rosacea.

How it Helps the Body's Esthetics

CBD oil is amazing for the overall esthetics of the body, including the hair. Hair needs vitamins and minerals, and often, if we don't get enough of them, we experience problems with the way hair and body looks.

For example, vitamins E and C can protect hair from split ends, thus reducing visible damage. The B vitamins help reconstruct hair; and if hair loss is imminent, you should use more B vitamins. CBD oil has these essential vitamins and nutrients, and more. Vitamins A and D are responsible for hair repair, creating a shinier look.

Then there is acne, a common problem that many people have deal with. It's mostly caused by too much sebum, meaning that lipid production is too high. Acne causes inflammation and blemishes on the face and is quite unsightly. CBD oil works with other oils in the body, controlling how much is produced. It targets the lipids in skin cells and is a preventative measure for acne, since it can be used to regulate sebum.

CBD oil is a great antibacterial agent and can target acne pimples directly. These are technically an infection on the face, and if treated with CBD, there won't be any more acne in the future. Eczema is treatable with CBD oil, which improves its appearance. As mentioned, the oil controls the immune response. It is the same with acne, a bacterium to which the immune system responds. CBD oil can control the response to the bacteria, and the inflammation that results, eliminating both instantly.

Using CBD oil can also help other skin conditions. Since CBD oil impacts the proliferation and differentiation of cells, it can be used to stop some kinds of skin cancer and allergic reactions. It works directly on a variety of dermatological problems such as blemishes, moles, and warts--in many cases preventing future instances. CBD oil can be used as alternative treatments for skin cancer patients when all others have failed.

Reducing Aging

How can CBD help reduce aging? Is it the fountain of youth? The endocannabinoid system is one of the greatest producers of basal cells. It grows all of the new cells when the old ones slough off. Accelerating the process creates younger-looking and more radiant skin.

CBD oil does this by means of vitamins, omega-3, and many antioxidants. It can protect the skin and increase its elasticity; it will stop free radicals from forming lines and wrinkles on the body.

CBD oil is clearly a great health and beauty addition, and you can use it in the form of skin creams, lotions, and facial washes. It has proven to be quite helpful to the body and can treat many skin conditions.

CHAPTER 6

Cooking with CBD

While the many uses of CBD oil are well known, not everyone knows that it can be used in cooking. Cooking is one of the easiest ways to make sure the recommended amount is obtained every day. Additionally, it can be a great addition to a dish. This chapter discusses why you should consider cooking with CBD whenever possible.

Using it in Edibles

Using CBD oil in food is safe. Consider cooking with it if you're struggling to take it each day.

Making your own edibles allows you to choose how much you want to include of the oil and other ingredients. Keep in mind that CBD oil is a fat soluble. It won't dissolve in water, but will in fat. This determines what you can make with it. Soups or watery food won't do since the oil won't mix properly. The easiest way to use CBD oil is in premixed cooking oil or butter.

While store-bought butter and oils loaded with CBD oil are convenient, it can also be homemade. Here's a recipe for butter:

1) Melt some butter and add the CBD oil.
2) Let the mixture simmer on a low setting. CBD has a boiling point of 320 degrees. Continue until the butter begins to bubble.
3) Store in a container until needed.

Mix with other oils like ghee, coconut oil, peanut butter, olive oil, or more. The choices are endless.

It's important not to overdo the oil in recipes as it can be overpowering or result in an overdose of certain vitamins and minerals. The dosage depends on the serving size and the amount a recipe call for. For instance, if you're baking six cookies, multiply the dosage by six, and that's how much is needed.

Know how many milligrams are in a cup of butter, or half a cup. Typically, a cup of CBD butter is about 10,000 mg with 5,000 mg for half a cup. Make sure it's divided evenly, so you know how much CBD is in each serving. The oil is easy to measure and is flavorless. It won't leave a strange taste.

Tips for Cooking with CBD Oil

When you begin working with CBD oil, it can be quite hard at first. Here are a few tips to remember when cooking:

- ✓ Make sure the CBD oil is from a good supplier. Buy high-quality oil for its potency and all the needed vitamins and minerals.
- ✓ Be mindful of the recipes you're using. Make sure they contain fat and oil for the CBD oil to mix well.
- ✓ CBD oil can be mixed with liquor. This actually does work if you're cooking something with vodka or rum in it. Make sure it isn't water-based since it won't mix with the oil.

Try an experimental batch to see if it works. Don't overdo the dosage of CBD, but if you do end up doing that, write down what you put in there and rectify it in the future. Watch where the CBD oil is stored as it is sensitive to light and heat. The last thing you want is to cook amazing food only to find out that it has been compromised because the CBD oil was left exposed. Make sure to store it in a dark and cool place. You can use the fridge, but make sure the light inside doesn't get left on since it can affect the overall nature of the product.

Remember, take the amount right for you. Say you have about 1,000 mg of oil and want to make twenty brownies. You're going to end up using 50 mg of the CBD oil, which might be too high. In most cases, half or even a quarter of that can make a world of a difference.

Note that a little goes a long way. You don't need to make a ton of butter to have a small set of edibles. Due to the lipids in CBD, it'll only bind to a certain number of cannabinoids. If you're using too much CBD oil, you're being wasteful. Make sure you follow the directions so you're not throwing too much out.

With this in mind, you'll be able to make some amazing edibles with this product. They work well in treating various ailments, and they are what many people turn to when looking for an alternative to cannabis products with THC. CBD oil doesn't create bad effects psychologically in a person, and it is a powerful form of healing. You won't get high by adding it to food; instead it will give you more nutrients, which is why it's encouraged to cook with CBD.

CHAPTER 7

How to Use CBD with Animals and at Home

CBD oil is a great addition to most health and wellness routines, but can it be used with pets? Is it safe to keep around pets? This is a question many pet owners ask because they don't want to hurt their furry friends. We'll now go into detail on how to use CBD oil with animals and any precautions that need to be taken.

Can I Use it With my Pets?

CBD oil can be used on pets and is approved by the FDA. However, you need to be careful since some oils don't contain the full content and might not help the pet. But remember, pets possess an endocannabinoid system, too, and can benefit from CBD used properly.

The oil helps to control the regulative processes in the animal's body similar to how it helps humans, whether it be our appetite, sleep, and/or overall metabolism. CBD oil isn't toxic either; and since it doesn't contain THC, it can be tolerated by animals. There are no psychoactive effects from ingestion.

For dogs, it helps with low energy, separation anxiety, eating problems, wound healing, and excessive barking. It can help with vet trips to calm pets down, and may prevent cancer, spasms, seizures, and arthritis. It helps with recovery and relaxation, too. It is great to give to a dog with high-anxiety, and those scared of noises or are aggressive toward humans.

It does many of the same things for cats if they're being introduced to new pets in the household, have issues with eating, are continually hiding or just have general fear of the litterbox. It helps stop eating weird stuff and if they're crying for no reason. Plus, it can help make vet trips and environmental changes easier to cope with. It's also great for reducing aggressiveness to other animals.

CBD is hard to overdose on, so you don't have to worry about this. It won't get the animal high, nor does it have anything in it that will cause bad side effects.

How to Administer CBD Oil to Pets

When it comes to pets, you can give them CBD in the form of an extract with a dropper placed in their food, through a treat, rubbed topically, or on their paws since they'll use their tongues to taste it and introduce it into their bodies. You can even get biscuits, capsules and caps, and even healing ointments if you want to try different products.

When administering the oil, you want to make sure that you don't give too much since it can be a bit shocking. Dosage varies with the situation, and you can experiment as you like. The rule of thumb is a 1 to 5 mg based on about 10-pounds of weight. For instance, cats are around 1 to 5 mg. For dogs, it varies. A 20-pound dog will be approximately 2 to 10 mg. For a dog that's 80-pounds or more, give around 8 to 40 mg.

You want to give the oil to pets at the lowest possible dose. A change will be noticed in about a half hour. Increase the dosage if a change in the pet isn't apparent. It may take a couple of treatments before there are marked differences.

If the animal is in pain, give the dose every eight hours. If the animal is taking CBD for behavioral issues, dose them a couple times a day, if needed. If changes are present after one dose, then dose them once a day. There isn't a table or set rule for this; supervise when dosing to see what changes are happening. Animals cannot overdose on CBD oil.

Precautions

There aren't any big precautions to worry about. Regulate the dosage and observe the animal behavior's for a couple of days. Always make sure that you're using safe and legal CBD products, because CBD oil doesn't have THC, which is toxic, so give them what they need.

If an animal has digested THC, rush them to the vet ER immediately.

As a precautionary, watch out for unknown CBD products as they may contain traces of chocolate, nuts, and xylitol. It is highly recommended to administer the oil in their food rather than buying products pre-mixed with the oil.

There have only been two cases of dogs dying while taking CBD. The cases were published in *The Journal of Veterinary Emergency and Critical Care* (2012). There were traces of chocolate in the product, and the dogs died of asphyxiation from their vomit. If buying pre-mixed products, research the company and ingredients before buying to prevent such an incident.

Make sure to store pre-mixed products or CBD oil, whichever you choose to use, away from animals. This way they cannot get the product and eat it. Even though CBD oil isn't toxic to animals, it does shock their bodies, creating more issues.

Here are a couple recipes for dog treats using CBD oil:

Peanut Butter Frozen Yogurt Dog Treat

Ingredients:

- About 32 ounces of vanilla yogurt
- CBD oil, enough for 2 drops per treat
- Cup of peanut butter

Directions:

1) In a microwave-safe bowl, combine the oil, yogurt, and peanut butter.
2) In an ungreased muffin pan lined with cupcake papers, pour mixture into units.
3) Freeze for about one hour or until completely frozen. Your furry friend and you can enjoy together!

CBD oil Doggy Treats

Ingredients:

- About two cups whole wheat flour or oats
- 1/3 cup peanut butter
- A tablespoon of 99% CBD coconut oil
- A mashed ripe banana

Directions:

1) Preheat the oven to 325°.
2) While it heats up, take about 8 tablespoons of coconut oil with a gram of the CBD oil, or just a tablespoon of the oil if it's already infused.
3) Blend the oats until a thick consistency, or use flour mixed with the banana, CBD coconut oil, and peanut butter. Mix until moist.
4) Put on a surface with some flour and shape into a small circle.

5) Use a cookie cutter and cut the treats out; and put them on a cookie sheet.

6) Bake until golden-brown, about 25-30 minutes. You should have about 30 treats, or 15 if you made them bigger.

CHAPTER 8

Side Effects of CBD, Dosing, and Where You Can Get It

It's important to know about the side effects of CBD oil and be prepared for them. If CBD oil has a specific dose, it's important to know about it. Maybe you're someone who wants to use CBD oil but has no idea where to buy it. Fortunately, these questions will all be answered in this chapter, and you'll know where to get good CBD oil.

Side Effects to Worry About

CBD oil produces some side effects, and it's good to know about them before you take the plunge. Unlike products that contain THC such as marijuana, it doesn't have the psychoactive issues that typically happen to those who take medical marijuana. CBD doesn't have the euphoric feeling that marijuana can produce.

Typically, CBD regulates the body, naturally changing a few of the above-mentioned negative effects. This will be the main reaction you will notice. You may use higher dosages for about four weeks for short-term care; and for long-term usage, take 300 mg every day.

Some people have noticed dry mouth, lightheadedness, drowsiness, and low blood pressure. However, there isn't much evidence to support this claim. Rather, the oil helps regulate blood pressure, body temperature, glucose and pH levels, heart rate, oxygen usage and carbon dioxide production, red blood cell generation, vomiting, metabolism, and electrolyte levels.

What's the Ideal Dose?

With CBD oil, the biggest thing to remember is that everyone is different and there isn't any universal point of reference. Typically, start with 25 mg and increase your intake by about 25 mg each week until the effects settle in. You should only go up to the point where you're getting the desired level.

The thing with CBD oil is that people must realize that each brands has different production standards, so follow the suggested 25 mg increase as CBD concentrations vary based on how they're prepared by the manufacturer. Here is a list of common dosages for a variety of issues, but always consult with your doctor or physician before starting any treatment:

- If taking CBD oil for appetite issues, only use about 1 mg for 6 weeks.
- For chronic pain, use between 2.5 to 20 mg for twenty-five days, or until your doctor tells you otherwise.
- For epilepsy, take 200 to 300 mg in the mouth daily for up to six months.
- If you're dealing with movement issues, take about 10 mg for each kilogram for about 6 weeks.
- For sleep disorders, take between 40 to 160 mg orally for the duration of the issue.
- For multiple sclerosis, take between 2.5 to 120 mg for about eight weeks. Do <u>NOT</u> take this with a THC combination.
- For glaucoma, take about 20 to 40 mg underneath the tongue. If taking over 40 mg, it may cause eye pressure issues.

- For schizophrenia, take between 40 to 1,280 mg orally, every day.

Dosing Cautions

Even a good thing needs to be supervised with caution. If you go over the suggested dosage amount or suggested time span, you can experience side effects in certain areas of the body. For instance, treating glaucoma with CBD can cause pressure on the eye if taken in a dose of over 40 mg a day.

Furthermore, everyone's body reacts differently to CBD oil. Our receptors are based on our gender, age, genetics, and general health. Whether you're using it to help treat a temporary concern or a chronic daily issue, it's important to remember that each person's tolerance is unique. If you're in prime health, you might not take as much as someone who have severe medical issues.

When it comes to expectant mothers or those breastfeeding, it might be best to avoid the oil unless you talk to your doctor.

If you have Parkinson's disease, taking high dosages might cause movement issues, and even tremors.

If you're going to use a spray underneath the tongue, you can do about 2.5 mg for 2 weeks.

Ideally, stay around 300 mg if you're going to be using higher amounts long term. You can safely take up to 1,500 mg for about 4 weeks before any side effects start to occur.

Currently, there aren't any known adverse effects, and the oil can be taken at high dosages; but if you're going to do this as a supplemental therapy, go with the lowest potency at first and work up to the proper level. Get a general idea of how much you may need each day, and then begin with this dose. Start with a few drops and gradually work up based on how you feel. Once you've figured out the ideal amount you need, determine whether you want to stay at that level or increase the dose. You'll soon be able to understand which serving works best for you.

If you're still having issues with the right dosage, see a doctor who specializes in CBD treatments and get the answers you need.

Where do you get it?

Since the oil is legal globally, you can buy it virtually anywhere. However, before you buy, consider a few factors:

- ✓ The size of the bottle
- ✓ The company reputation
- ✓ Any reports of it being diluted or issues from customers
- ✓ Whether you want to take it as a tincture, concentration, vape, or any other way
- ✓ The right strength of CBD oil you need
- ✓ All ingredients are listed and know what they are

You should know that various products come in different forms, sizes, and shapes. Make sure you buy the right level of CBD oil. You can't get too much, but knowing how much you need will help you get the right kind. Make sure the bottle or ingredient says CBD oil and not hemp oil, as they may sometimes use the latter instead.

If you get pure CBD oil, you'll be getting it fully from the hemp oil plant itself. You should, however, think about the concentration and your budget. Certain products provide a little bit or a lot, and that's a huge factor. The purer the oil, the more it will cost ($200-400/bottle).

There are tinctures or liquid extracts you can take under the tongue. CBD tinctures tend to use natural ingredients and come at a discounted price. The tinctures vary from 100-500 mg/bottle.

The CBD oil can come as a vaporizer as well. This is a newer way of taking CBD as it enters the lungs directly, allowing the body to absorb it faster and better. Plus, it is a cheaper alternative than the pure oil ($35/each).

If you're going to be using it for the body for rejuvenation, creams or moisturizers are a great way to do so. They're about $25/each and usually contain about 50 mg of CBD oil per use; plus, it also comes with other important nutrients and essential oils. These are definitely helpful additions if you're looking to improve your body.

CBD-infused body washes and hair products can be bought. You can use these products as a part of your basic hygiene as they are infused with vitamins, fatty acids, CBD oil and other great supplements. Including these items in your bodily routine will be beneficial and you will have amazing results.

Remember to always do your research before buying any product from any company. It's hard to find a reliable company since CBD oil is relatively new and has only recently become popular. Moreover, company reviews will tell you everything you need to know about the oil and the results of other consumers' usage like allergic and other reactions.

When choosing a product, make sure that all ingredients are marked on the packaging or bottle, and that nothing questionable is included. It should also have storage, user information, serving size, and expiration date, along with side effects, if any. You should be able to clearly see these before buying.

Buy can capsules and other supplementary forms. Many people prefer them. However, any product has the downside of not being as pure. Research the brand before purchasing.

Many times with CBD oil, you may need a prescription to purchase it. But there are over-the-counter products you can buy online. If you want to medically treat various conditions, you will have to go to a doctor and try other treatments before you can obtain the CBD oil.

CHAPTER 9

Recipes That Use CBD Oil

And now at last, recipes. While we touched on how you can cook with CBD oil, it's important to know a few recipes that will help you get the full benefit of CBD oil easily. This chapter will provide some fun recipes that use CBD oil with, and how you can get enjoy this remarkable oil.

Cinnamon CBD Parfait with Hemp Milk

Serves: 2
Prep time: 5 mins
Cook time: 6-8 hours

Ingredients:

- 2 cups of either regular milk or hemp milk (the hemp milk is optional, but you might like the extra benefits)
- 1/3 cup agave nectar
- ½ teaspoon vanilla
- 1/3 cup chia seeds
- .33 grams of 99% Pure CBD powder

Directions:

1) Take all the ingredients save the chia seeds and mix them in a blender. Keep it on the highest setting for a minute until all mixed together
2) Put the blender contents into a bowl with the chia seeds. Mix until it reaches a pudding consistency.

3) Add the pudding mixture to an airtight container and cool for at least 6-8 hours until the seeds become gelatin-like.
4) Mix the mixture a few times within the first hour to keep it the pudding consistency, if needed.
5) Add your favorite fruit. Serve.

CBD Carrot Cake

Serves: 4
Prep time: 25 mins
Cooking time: 60 mins

Ingredients:

- 1 greased cake pan
- 1 teaspoon soda for baking
- 1 ¼ teaspoons of salt, finely grained
- 1 cup of buttermilk
- 3 eggs
- 2 cups of flour
- 2 teaspoons of ground cinnamon
- 2 tablespoons vegetable oil mixed with CBD oil
- 2 teaspoons vanilla
- 1 cup of coconut flakes
- 1 cup raisins
- ¾ cups sugar
- 2 cups of cut carrots
- 1 cup chopped walnuts

For the frosting:

- A beater or mixer
- 1 teaspoon vanilla
- 1 cup of cream cheese
- A cup of soft butter

-   4 cups of fine powdered sugar

Directions:

1) Preheat oven to 375°.
2) Put the dry ingredients in a bowl and mix well.
3) Put the wet ingredients in the eggs and combine.
4) Mix the wet and dry ingredients together.
5) Add the fruits and nuts together in a different bowl and mix.
6) Mix the batter with the fruits and nuts and bake for about an hour, or until you get a clean toothpick.
7) Cool. Then make the frosting mixture.
8) Frost the cake and cool. Cut it up and serve.

Cranberry Sauce

Servings: 8
Prep time: 5 mins
Cook time: 45 mins

Ingredients:

-   1 pound of chopped strawberries
-   2 tablespoons CBD oil
-   1/3 cup raw honey
-   ½ cup orange juice
-   1 pinch sea salt
-   1 ½ tablespoons cornstarch

Directions:

1) Take all the ingredients excluding the OJ, salt, and cornstarch, and cook on medium-low heat.
2) Combine cornstarch and OJ in a separate bowl.
3) Add it to the pan and mix together until it thickens. About 8-10.

4) Take it off the heat, adding the salt, and cool at room temperature. It will thicken.
5) Pour it over your favorite dish or serve with turkey.

Fig soda Bread with Cherries and CBD

Serves: 12
Prep time: 20 mins
Cook time: 40 mins

Ingredients:

- 2 cups of organic all-purpose flour
- ½ cup organic oats
- 2 tablespoons CBD oil tincture
- 1 cup whole wheat flour
- ¼ cup hemp seeds
- 1 teaspoon salt
- 1 teaspoon baking soda
- 1 egg
- 1 teaspoon baking powder
- 1 cup of buttermilk
- ½ cup of Monterey cherries kept whole
- ½ cup chopped figs

Directions:

1) Preheat oven to 375° and line a baking sheet with parchment paper.
2) Mix the flours, oats, salt, hemp seeds, soda, and baking powder together in a bowl.
3) Pour wet ingredients into another bowl and add the flour mixture. Continue to stir until it becomes a dough.
4) Add the cherries and figs. Mix.
5) Knead the dough into a ball and place on the baking sheet.

6) Using your forearms, flatten the dough. With a paring knife, score the dough.
7) Bake for about 40 minutes, or until it sounds hollow if you touch the bottom
8) Cool on a baking rack for 30 minutes. Serve.

Peanut Butter Chocolate Bars

Serves: 16
Prep time: 15 mins
Cooking time: 20-25 or so minutes

Ingredients:

- ½ cup vegetable oil
- 1 teaspoon vanilla
- 1 cup brown sugar
- ½ cup CBD-infused oil, either vegetable, corn, or canola
- 1 egg
- 1 cup chocolate chips
- 1/3 cup peanut butter
- 1 cup flour

Directions:

1) Preheat oven to 350º. Add oil on the baking pan and set aside.
2) Add the CBD oil to the mixture: egg, brown sugar, peanut butter, and vanilla extract in a bowl.
3) Add the flour and mix well. Pour into the baking pan and spread evenly.
4) Top with chocolate chips.
5) Bake for 20 minutes or until done.
6) Cool for 30 minutes. Cut into bars. Serve.

These are great cool or warm!

With CBD oil recipes, it is often a matter of the same thing: just add the CBD before you begin. Try adding CBD to other recipes you like. Just be cautious about how much you use, and make sure the food isn't water-based. If you're looking to cook with CBD oil, try following these recipes. They will help you go on your own and get on the right track to food with added benefits for your body.

CHAPTER 10

21-day Challenge

Many individuals are turning to CBD oil for different reasons. As you have read, it's quite different from marijuana and other cannabis products; and since it doesn't have the same effects as THC on the body, people are looking to CBD for health and wellness solutions.

You have seen how it can help the body from boosting mood to treating the symptoms of breast cancer, and more. It's remarkable that it can do so much, and you can use it in so many different ways from skincare to cooking. Plus, it doesn't have a ton of side effects.

For an added benefit, we've included a few recipes to begin your adventure. Next time you cook, add CBD oil to other dishes and you will know exactly how much to use for non-water-based meals.

Take your next step by joining the 21-day challenge. This challenge will have you using CBD oil every day. Use it in your face cleanser or other skincare products, cook with it or taking a couple of drops under the tongue to get into the habit of using the oil. You'll notice immediately how much calmer and happier you feel with just a few steps. Yes, it does work that fast.

The 21-day challenge is simple. For 21 days, use the oil. Try to cook with it or use it in your daily body care routines. Use the recommended dosage given on the bottle, or if you have a condition described in Chapter 9, use it specifically for that. After 21 days, record the difference and you see how CBD oil has helped you. You can do the challenge for longer of course. Many have done it for 90 days, and they've seen a huge a difference in their lives. If you're thinking about doing it, the first thing you should do is sit down and establish some goals. Choose something simple and attainable that will help you create a better and more enhanced form of you.

From here, once you have an idea of the process, it's important to get an oil that fits your routine. Look at the dosages, and you'll be able to find the one that best meets your needs. From then on, use the magic oil every single day.

Typically, about a drop or two can make a world of a difference whether you use the oil in a face and skin cleanser once a day, or even cook a meal with it. You should definitely journal every single day, acknowledging what's happening in your body; and from there, you will see for yourself the changes that the challenge has made.

The 21-day challenge is something you can work on yourself, and if you really want to see a difference in your life, try recording the mental effects as well. Now you can go in knowing in advance the many great benefits; and if you record everything that happens, you'll understand the potential that CBD oil has to offer for your both personal and mental health too. Take control of your health and wellness today with CBD oil, and you'll never be the same.

REVIEWS

Reviews and feedback help improve this book and the author. If you enjoy this book, we would greatly appreciate it if you were able to take a few moments to share your opinion and post a review.

www.ingramcontent.com/pod-product-compliance
Lightning Source LLC
Chambersburg PA
CBHW050632190326
41458CB00008B/2236

.